A Book of Practical Diabetes Health & Prevention

Text Copyright © Extensive Enterprises Corp.

All rights reserved. No part of this guide may be reproduced in any form without permission in writing from the publisher except in the case of brief quotations embodied in critical articles or reviews.

Legal & Disclaimer

The information contained in this book and its contents is not designed to replace or take the place of any form of medical or professional advice; and is not meant to replace the need for independent medical, financial, legal or other professional advice or services, as may be required. The content and information in this book have been provided for educational and entertainment purposes only.

The content and information contained in this book have been compiled from sources deemed reliable, and it is accurate to the best of the Author's knowledge, information, and belief. However, the Author cannot guarantee its accuracy and validity and cannot be held liable for any errors and/or omissions. Further, changes are periodically made to this book as and when needed. Where appropriate and/or necessary, you must consult a professional (including but not limited to your doctor, attorney, financial advisor or such other professional advisor) before using any of the suggested remedies, techniques, or information in this book.

Upon using the contents and information contained in this book, you agree to hold harmless the Author from and against any damages, costs, and expenses, including any legal fees potentially resulting from the application of any of the information provided by this book. This disclaimer applies to any loss, damages or injury caused by the use and application, whether directly or indirectly, of any advice or information presented, whether for breach of contract, tort, negligence, personal injury, criminal intent, or under any other cause of action.

You agree to accept all risks of using the information presented inside this book.

You agree that by continuing to read this book, where appropriate and/or necessary, you shall consult a professional (including but not limited to your doctor, attorney, or financial advisor or such other advisor as needed) before using any of the suggested remedies, techniques, or information in this book.

Table of Contents

Introduction 1

Chapter 1: What is Diabetes? 4

    The History of Diabetes as A Disease 4

    A Few Facts About Diabetes 6

        Diabetes Type 2...7

        Diabetes Type 1...8

    Where We Are Today 9

    Who Is at Risk for Diabetes? 10

        For Diabetes Type 2..10

        For Diabetes Type 1..12

    The associated complications 13

        Cardiovascular diseases 13

        Neuropathy 13

        Eye damage 14

        Kidney damage...14

        Alzheimer's disease..15

        Preeclampsia 15

    What can be done? 15

        Physical activity 15

Diet 16

Change your habits 16

Chapter 2: Why It Is Important to Manage Your Diabetes? 18

Diabetes and The Quality of Life 18

Safe Diabetes Levels 19

Microvascular Diseases 20

    Retinopathy 20

    Nephropathy 21

    Neuropathy 21

Macrovascular Diseases 22

    Cardiovascular diseases 22

Benefits of a Healthy Lifestyle 22

    Increased immunity 23

    Increased energy 23

    Weight loss 23

    Improved mood and mental health 23

When to see the Doctor 24

Chapter 3: How Is Diabetes Typically Controlled? 26

Controlling Diabetes Naturally Through Diet 27

    What to eat? 27

    What not to eat 33

Controlling Diabetes Naturally Through Exercise.........37

    Great Exercises...38

    Tips for working out 41

Managing Through Medication.......................................42

Chapter 4: Why Managing Diabetes Naturally is Preferred 47

Why you should consider the natural remedies 47

The Alternative Therapies 49

    Physical intervention 49

    The herbal medicines 51

    Dietary supplements...57

Chapter 5: Choosing a Diet to Help You Control Your Diabetes 61

Some of the eating habits 62

    Eating while hungry 62

    Judging the food by taste 62

    Buying the food based on the price tag.......................63

    Eating with your emotions..63

    Eating while watching television.................................64

    Conforming to the social convention 64

    Sleep eating..64

    Not paying attention to what you eat 65

Rushing through time 65
Improving your diets 65
Factors to consider when choosing a diet 66
    Dietary requirements for managing diabetes naturally 67
    Allergies 69
    Religion 69
    The cost of the food 70
    Your activity level 70
    Consider the benefits and side effects 70
    Preferences 71
Types of diets to choose from 72
    G.I Diets 73
    Pritikin diets 75
    Vegan Diets 77
    Paleo diets 78
    Low-carb diets 80
Tips for making the meal tasty 82
    Replace the solid fats with liquid oils 82
    Replace the high-fat dairy 82
    Experiment with flavors 83

Chapter 6: Diets in Detail 84

The types of diets 84

    Mediterranean diets 84

    Ketogenic diets 87

    Atkins Diet 91

    Vegetarian diet 94

    The South Beach Diet 97

Chapter 7: Exercises to Help You Lose Weight 99

Three Body Types 99

    Ectomorph 99

    Mesomorph 100

    Endomorph 100

General weight loss exercises 101

    Cardio exercises 101

    Walking 102

    Cycling 103

    Elliptical exercises 103

    Swimming 103

    Jumping rope exercises 104

    Stair climber exercises 104

    Rowing exercises 104

    HIIT 105

    Kettlebells 105

    Sprinting 105

    Jogging 106

    Stretching and balance exercises 106

    Strength training 110

    Barbell exercises 112

    Dumbbell exercises 113

Chapter 8: Getting in the Right Mindset to Maintain Healthy Diabetes Levels 114

    How to prepare mentally 114

        Get a dietician 115

        Set your goals 115

        Mental visualization 117

        Have a detailed plan 118

        Get support 118

        Positive affirmations 119

        Replace your bad habits 120

        Be patient 120

        Reward yourself 121

    Developing Self-discipline 121

        Time management 122

        Creates stability 122

- Builds inner strength 123
- Helps you to control your appetite and cravings 123
- How to develop self-discipline 123
  - Define what you want 124
  - What are the changes that you need to make? 124
  - Find a role model 125
  - Identify your habits 125
  - Identify your triggers 125
  - Develop a plan 126
  - Accountability 126
- Sources of support 126
  - Family and friends 127
  - Support groups 127
  - Your healthcare team 127
  - Online communities 128

Conclusion 129
- Choose the right diet 129
- Choose the right exercise routine 130
- Consider the alternatives 130
- Develop self-discipline and the right mindset 131
- Don't do it alone 131

Introduction

If you choose to read this book, most probably you or someone else close to you is facing problems with blood sugar levels. It might be that your previous fasting blood sugar levels are higher than the normal range – which could be in the prediabetes range of 100-125mg/dL (milligrams per deciliter) indicating that you have a weakened tolerance and are at risk of developing diabetes. If your fasting blood glucose reaches more than 125mg/dL, you are already in the onset for type 2 diabetes.

Some of your test results might be showing your hemoglobin AIC levels which measure your average blood sugar over the previous several months are prominent – meaning they were either between 5.5% to 6.5%, the threshold for diabetes and higher than 6.5% telling you that you may actually have diabetes.

Knowing that your blood sugar levels are too elevated can be baffling and upsetting. The fact that both prediabetes and type 2 diabetes are a precursor for developing diabetes itself, these also tend to develop slowly over many years. Many of us think that once you have been diagnosed with either of these conditions, there is nothing you can do but to take diabetes medication and hope that someday it will go away. As a diabetes writer and researcher, I want you to feel assured that there are always steps you can do to improve your body's response to insulin and to normalize your metabolism to eliminate those unwanted sugar spikes in your blood from the moment you read this book today.

This simple motivation has insightful implications. This means that if you have prediabetes, you can prevent your condition from progressing to diabetes or possibly even reverse everything back to normal levels. If you already have type 2 diabetes, you can still improve significantly your body's natural sugar levels and gradually reduce, and in some cases even eliminate – your need for synthetic insulin, metformin, and other diabetes medication.

The promise of A Book of Practical Diabetes Health & Prevention is simple. If you read and follow everything written in this book, you will begin seeing improvements in your body in terms of metabolizing your blood glucose levels. With the proper diet, exercise and natural medications, you'll become more relaxed, lose weight and become more fit. Your overall health will improve as your balanced immune system fights off unwanted risks to your body.

Chapter 1:

What is Diabetes?

Did you know that Diabetes is a deadly disease? It is the 7th leading cause of death in the world. Diabetes is a pandemic that has swept America and the world at large by storm. The condition has become more rampant today in the 21st Century affecting both young and old. Over the decades, the assumption has been that diabetes is a disease for the affluent. But, contrary to that, reports have indicated even middle and low-income people are prone to diabetes.

The History of Diabetes as A Disease

What is known today as Diabetes mellitus carried a different name a couple of centuries ago? In the medieval ages, diabetes was an incurable disease and a death sentence to many due to the lack of treatment. Diabetes is characterized by the inability of the body to process sugar. Matthew Dobson was the first to observe this in 1776 when he confirmed the 'sweet urine' produce by diabetic patients was sugar.

Between 980 and 1037, Persia Avicenna collected data and provided a detailed report on the disease. Among the symptoms that he noted included the decline in appetite, the excretion of sweet urine, and the decline in sexual activity. He was the first to describe the exact condition- diabetes. Persia provided a record of the disease's characteristic in general, however, in the 18th and 19th century a distinction between the different types of diabetes was done. Johann Peter Frank was the first to distinguish between diabetes Mellitus and diabetes insipidus.

In 1889, Joseph Von Mering made a significant discovery- he identified the role that the pancreas plays in regulating Diabetes. Research carried out on dogs indicated that the dog breeds that had their pancreas removed presented all the symptoms associated with diabetes. Later in 1910, Sir Edward Albert noted that diabetes was caused by lack of insulin in the body.

The discovery of the cause of diabetes led to the introduction of the treatments. In 1919, Dr. Fredrick introduced a therapy that would manage the disease- dieting and starvation.

While the diet restriction was a solution, the scientists wanted a more permanent solution to the condition which led to the discovery of insulin as a treatment. Sir Fredrick Grant and his partner Charles Herbert demonstrated that they could cure diabetes. They echoed the work of Joseph Mering and Oskar Minkowski by attempting to reverse diabetes in the dogs. The two scientists used the insulin excreted from the cow's pancreas for their experiment. They later purified the hormone and made it effective to be used by humans. In 1922, the first trial was carried out and Leonard Thompson, 14 years of age, was the first recipient. He lived for 13 years after the injection of insulin but succumbed to pneumonia at the age of 27.

Sir Harold Percival made the distinction between diabetes type 1 and type 2 in 1937.

A Few Facts About Diabetes

Diabetes is a silent disease whose symptoms are ferocious. However, as aggressive as the symptoms might be, their simplicity leads to the inaction of most people who have it. As a result, many people remain undiagnosed. The condition is characterized by increased hunger, urination, fatigue, blurred vision, and excessive thirst.

Over the years, scientists have tried to make a distinction between the different types of diabetes.

Diabetes Type 2

It is the most common type amongst the adult generation today, and it is lifestyle related. While overweight people are more prone to the condition, diabetes mellitus can occur to all. Most overweight and obese people have diabetes, but not all diabetic patients are overweight.

Diabetes type 2 is caused by the inability of the body to utilize the insulin produced. In the severe cases, the pancreas stops the production of the insulin altogether due to high levels of cholesterol. With the inability of the body to process the glucose into energy, the sugar is absorbed into the bloodstream leading to the above-mentioned symptoms.

Since diabetes type 2 is lifestyle related, medical professionals recommend diet regulation and exercise to control the condition naturally when possible. There are, however, a few cases that may warrant the use of insulin to manage the disease.

Diabetes Type 1

The primary cause of the condition is unknown. However, research reports have indicated that low immunity can be a trigger. Low immunity translates to the failure of the body to fight bacteria and other viruses which in turn lead to the destruction of the insulin cells. Diabetes type 1 is a genetic disease. But, its onset can be triggered by environmental factors and lifestyle. Diabetes type 1 patients solely depend on insulin in combination with good nutrition to manage the condition.

The other types of diabetes include gestational diabetes and pre-diabetes. Pre-diabetes can go unnoticed because it presents no symptoms. However, with regular visits to the doctor, early detection can be achieved. The progression of the condition to diabetes is inevitable, and if left untreated it can cause major havoc in your life. However, with good diet and exercise, you can reverse blood sugar back to normal levels.

Where We Are Today

In the last couple of years, the prevalence of diabetes has significantly increased. In today's world teenagers and young adults are among some of the worst affected.

The National Diabetes Statistics Report, 2017 indicated that 30.3 million people who are about 9.4% of the population are living with diabetes in the United States. Approximately 7.2 million people are undiagnosed.

Diabetes is not only a deadly disease; it is costly as well. The direct and indirect cost of diabetes (diagnosed) was $ 245 billion in the United States in 2012 according to the report. The average medical expenditures were $ 13,700. When it comes to the death reports, approximately 79,535 deaths in 2015 were as a result of diabetes. These numbers are alarming considering we are in the 21st century. Great strides have been taken to address the gruesome reality of diabetes. However, a lot more needs to be done to lower the overall numbers. Creating awareness of the condition seems to be the one significant solution to the never-ending challenges.

Who Is at Risk for Diabetes?

For Diabetes Type 2

Diabetes type 2 is a lifestyle disease. While other preexisting factors can trigger the condition, lack of proper nutrition and exercise is the primary cause of the condition.

Overweight and obese

These people are at risk of getting the disease. The presence of cholesterol in the body can inhibit the utilization and also the production of insulin.

Sedentary lifestyle

Persons that have embraced an idle lifestyle have a higher risk of diabetes than those people who are moderately active.

Family history

Genetics play a significant role when it comes to diabetes. If your family has a history of diabetes, there is an increased chance that you may get it. Even though there is a likelihood that diabetes can come knocking at your door, you can avoid it. Proper nutrition and regular consultations will keep the disease at bay.

Older people

Age is a factor of consideration. The risk of diabetes increases as we age. Decrease exercise, muscle loss, and weight gain have been attributed to the increased risk.

Gestational diabetes

Mothers who experienced gestational diabetes when they were pregnant are at an increased risk of getting diabetes.

PCOS

Polycystic Ovary syndrome is a trigger for the condition. PCOS is increasingly becoming the norm among fertile women. The condition is categorized by irregular menstrual cycle, hair growth, and weight gain which can lead to obesity. These are conditions that can increase the risk of diabetes.

Persons with abnormal cholesterol and triglycerides

It is the assumption that abnormal cholesterol levels are only seen in obese and overweight people. However, unhealthy diets lead to the deposit of large amounts of cholesterol in the body. The abnormal levels of cholesterol are determined by the levels of low-density lipoprotein and high-density lipoprotein. The HDL, 'good' lipoproteins help to regulate the work of cholesterol in the body. Therefore, low levels of HDL increase the risk of diabetes.

For Diabetes Type 1

Genetics

If a parent or a sibling has the condition, the child or the young adult is at risk.

Compromised immunity

The presence of auto-antibodies in the body increases the risk of diabetes. These are the damaging immune cells that attack the insulin-producing cells. The auto-antibodies are no doubt a risk factor, but not all persons with the condition develop diabetes type 1.

Environment and geography

People who are exposed to viral diseases are prone to the condition. Countries like Sweden and Finland have a higher rate of diabetes type 1.

The associated complications

It is known that when diabetes comes knocking, it doesn't come alone. The complications associated with diabetes develop gradually. Most of the conditions can be avoided with proper management of diabetes. Some of the complications can be managed, and others are life-threatening and can lead to death.

Cardiovascular diseases

Diabetes significantly increases the risk of CVDs. Stroke, narrow arteries, and chest pains are the most common complications.

Neuropathy

Nerve damage characterizes the condition. The excess sugar in the bloodstream can cause tremendous damage to the capillaries. These blood vessels are responsible for blood circulation, especially to the legs. The effects of the nerve damage include a tingling sensation, numbness, pain and a burning feeling in the legs. The tingling feeling begins at the tip of the toes and fingers before advancing upwards. When the condition goes untreated, it can lead to erectile dysfunction in men, nausea, and vomiting.

Eye damage

Excessive blood sugar can damage the retina which causes blindness. The condition can also lead to the development of glaucoma or cataracts.

Kidney damage

A great percentage of the diabetic patients experience failure in one or both their kidneys. Kidneys play an essential part in the detoxification of the body. The organs contain glomeruli which filter waste material from the blood. The presence of sugar in the bloodstream can cause havoc to these important blood cells which can severely damage the organ or worse still cause the irreversible onset of kidney disease.

Alzheimer's disease

Failure to control the blood sugar can put you at risk of developing the condition.

Preeclampsia

The condition is defined by the increased in blood pressure, swelling of the feet, and abnormal levels of protein in the urine. It is only the pregnant mothers who experience preeclampsia. If left unchecked, diabetes can lead to life-threatening consequences for the mother and the unborn child.

What can be done?

Prevention is better than cure, and when it comes to diabetes, this statement holds true. There are various ways recommended by medical professionals that can significantly improve your overall diabetes health.

Physical activity

The term exercise frightens a lot of people and understandably so. But, going to the gym is not the only way to achieve your goal. You can choose to walk in nature, taking the stairs instead of elevators, parking your car far away so you can walk, and things like these are just some of the ways that you can incorporate exercise into your daily routine. The idea is to avoid leading a sedentary life.

Diet

Your diet can also impact your general wellness positively and negatively. Regulating your portions is a great place to start. Eating plenty of fiber and whole grains is essential. As a diabetic patient, luxury is not on your side, and it is important to consider eating foods that lower the blood sugar levels. Avoid foods like simple carbohydrates like white rice and bread. With these foods, you will become hyperglycemic in no time. Lean meat and white meat should be among your top diets.

Change your habits

Smoking is one of the factors that can increase the risk of diabetes. It is essential for you to quit smoking entirely to avoid the onset of diabetes. While alcohol has been linked to reducing the risk of diabetes, too much consumption can lead to serious consequences.

Diabetes type 2 is lifestyle related, and that means it can be avoided. But, if you are suffering from the condition, don't fear. A change in your lifestyle will help to control the blood sugar and get your blood sugar levels back to normal levels.

Chapter 2:

Why It Is Important to Manage Your Diabetes?

The desire for a happy and satisfied life is a commonality we all share. But, leading a stress-free life is at times a mirage especially to people living with diabetes. Diabetes is a burdensome disease that affects not only your health but your quality of life in general.

Diabetes and The Quality of Life

Most people enjoy the opportunity to eat what they want, but that is a luxury that diabetic people can't enjoy. Their day to day life is filled with concerns about the levels of their blood sugar. For people with diabetes, all extremes of the blood sugar levels (hypoglycemia and hyperglycemia) are problematic.

Diabetes comes with never-ending demands; from eating healthy to exercising. The disease also takes a toll on your family as well. Your family is forced to consider alternative lifestyles and foods that are suitable for you. The financial burden is also too much for most people to bear.

Diabetes co-exists with other chronic diseases that are a constant threat to most people. It is for that reason that you are advised to seek medical help in the management of the condition. Most people manage to control the disease. But, a small percentage of people with diabetes end up being clinically depressed especially if they are alone in this journey.

Safe Diabetes Levels

Because the onset of diabetes creates room for other diseases to creep in, it is important to learn how to manage the condition. Knowing the normal and safe levels of blood glucose will help in the long run.

- Fasting, 100 or less
- Before meals, 70 to 130
- After meals approximately 1 to 2 hours 180 or less
- Before exercise, if taking insulin, at least 100
- Bedtime, 100 to 140

The normal blood sugar includes: fasting blood sugar of about 180 about two hours after meals.

A1C levels at or around 7%

It is crucial for you to manage your diabetes. Failure to regulate the condition will lead to life-threatening illnesses that can dramatically shorten your life. The complications associated with diabetes are divided into two: macrovascular and microvascular.

Microvascular Diseases

Retinopathy

It is an eye disease triggered by the destruction of the retinal nerves. High blood sugar causes the nerves to become inactive leading to eye blindness, glaucoma, and cataracts. When you begin to experience blurred vision, it is your cue to visit the doctor.

Early detection of the condition can either prevent the onset of the eye blindness or delay it. Good metabolic control can help slow the progression of the disease.

Nephropathy

Kidney disease is prevalent among people living with diabetes. High blood sugar causes damage to the blood vessels that enable kidneys to function efficiently. The results include kidney disease which will eventually lead to kidney failure and ultimately death.

Early detection of the disease can prevent the progression of the condition. Dialysis and kidney transplant have proven to be long-term solutions. The management of kidney failure can be done through proper diet.

Neuropathy

Most of the diabetic patients have reported having nerve disease (not on the same level) at different times in their lives. Hyperglycemia causes failure of the capillaries that transport blood to your limbs. It also leads to the decrease of the blood flow. The nerve damage causes sensory loss, impotence in men and damage to your legs.

Numbness, tingling feeling, pain in your feet, and erectile dysfunction in men are some of the symptoms associated with the condition. If not treated early, neuropathy can lead to amputation.

Macrovascular Diseases

Cardiovascular diseases

High blood sugar leads to the onset of atherosclerosis. The clogging of the blood arteries leads to decreased blood flow affecting the functioning of the heart muscles. This can result in heart attack, stroke, and decreased immunity.

Early detection can delay the progression of the disease. However, dealing with the risk factors of the condition like smoking, hypertension, and cholesterol will help in regulating the situation.

Benefits of a Healthy Lifestyle

The complications mentioned above can scare anyone no doubt. But, there is still hope of redemption- diet and exercising. The one ticket to avoiding the difficulties and leading a healthy and happy life is to control your blood sugar. Changing your lifestyle altogether will go a long way in regulating your diabetes health and wellness.

In general, living a healthy lifestyle is beneficial to your life:

Increased immunity

With the change in environment, bacteria, and viruses have become a part of life. You need to have a healthy immune system to fight the diseases. Eating vitamin C rich foods will help in boosting your immunity.

Increased energy

We all need strength to carry out our daily activities. With regular exercises, you can increase your energy. It is advisable to eat nutrient-dense foods on a daily basis.

Weight loss

The prevalence of diabetes and other lifestyle diseases has increased, and it is time to take control of the situation. Eating healthy foods like vegetables and fruits in combination with exercise will promote weight loss.

Improved mood and mental health

Believe it or not, your feelings are largely based on what you eat. If you eat fatty foods, you will end up feeling drowsy and feel a decrease in your energy. The food you choose can also affect your concentration and your general mental health. It is essential for you to eat vitamin-rich foods to promote better memory and concentration.

When to see the Doctor

If you are pre-diabetic, the condition can go unnoticed because it presents no obvious symptoms. Only through regular checkups will you determine if you are becoming diabetic. If you begin to experience, fatigue, increased urination, and increased hunger, you need to visit the doctor to test for the early stages of diabetes.

When you are diagnosed with diabetes, you need to keep an eye on the levels of your blood glucose.

Blurring vision, trouble with sleep (you can't stay awake), deep and fast breathing, pain in your abdomen, nausea and vomiting, being confused, a burning and tingling sensation on the tips of your fingers and toes, and a fruity breath, are symptoms associated with diabetes. You need to see a doctor if you begin to experience any of these symptoms.

Diabetes is a demanding disease no doubt. But, with proper planning, exercise, support, and willpower, you can manage the disease and finally achieve the quality of life that you deserve.

Chapter 3:

How Is Diabetes Typically Controlled?

Being diagnosed with Diabetes can be stressful, but as complicated as the disease might be, you can beat it. You can live a fruitful and fulfilling life. The secret to attaining the quality of life that you want is controlling your blood sugar. As you know, diabetes is characterized by the inability of the body to either produce insulin or use its already available insulin. Regardless of the type of diabetes that you have, reducing the level of blood sugar in your bloodstream is the only way to manage the disease. Besides, controlling your blood sugar will also lower the risk of getting the associated diseases.

So, how do you keep diabetes at bay? It can be done through exercise, your diet, and medication. If you have diabetes Type 2, the combination of diet and exercise can do the trick. However, if the disease is progressing at an alarming rate, the doctors may prescribe medication to help you control it.

Controlling Diabetes Naturally Through Diet

What to eat?

Did you know that diabetes progresses in steps? Pre-diabetes is the first step. When you are pre-diabetic, you present no symptoms. But, without adequately addressing the blood sugar issue, the condition will progress into diabetes. It is for that reason that the doctors recommend consulting a dietician to help you plan your meals.

Sedentary life and unhealthy foods have been blamed for the development of diabetes Type 2. If you are diabetic, you need to adhere strictly to the diabetic diet designed for you.

A diabetic diet is composed of foods that are taken in moderate amounts. The purpose of the diet is to help you regulate blood sugar while at the same time getting your daily calorie requirement.

There are many diets that you can adapt to your daily life. But, simplicity is important in regulating your blood sugar and staying healthy. Don't go overboard in planning the diet. You may want to consider consulting a registered dietician to help design a suitable diet plan for you.

There are different ways that you can also ensure that you regulate your diet. The plat method is one perfect example. The American Diabetes Association has designed the plate method to help people plan their meals accordingly. Half of the plate should include vegetables, ¼ of the plate should be filled with protein and the other ¼ to have complex carbohydrates.

You can also use the exchange system to help in your diet planning. Counting calories (a tedious process) can also help you. You will, however, need to know the number of calories in a food group to plan effectively.

Carbohydrates

Knowing how much and what type of carbohydrates is important when you are managing your diabetes. You have to keep in mind that there should be a balance of how much insulin is in your body and the carbohydrates you take in making a difference on the levels of your blood glucose.

Foods that are rich in carbohydrates are the main source of energy, and thus they are important. But, there are two types of carbohydrates that you can choose from; complex carbohydrates and simple carbohydrates. When you eat your meal, the body will digest the sugars and convert them into glucose for easy absorption.

If you eat simple carbs (white rice, bread, potatoes), the glucose level will be elevated which leads to hyperglycemia. It is essential for you to opt for the complex carbohydrates (brown rice, whole wheat bread). These foods take longer to be digested, and they are absorbed slowly.

Moreover, exploring carbohydrates requires you to understand more the effect that they have on your blood sugar levels. To know how to keep your blood sugar levels within your target range, you should be able to use carb counting. This allows you to have more choices when planning your meals. It might seem complex but this only involves counting the number of carbohydrate grams in meals and matching it on your insulin dose. A right balance of carbs, physical activity and insulin can help you manage your sugar levels.

Also, you need to consider the glycemic index. There are specific diets that can help you manage diabetes. These will be discussed thoroughly in the next chapters. Another option that can be utilized as well is low-calorie sweeteners.

These are also called artificial sweeteners which can be used to sweeten some of your food and beverages as a replacement for sugar.

Best Choices

- ✓ Whole grains, such as brown rice, oatmeal, and quinoa
- ✓ Baked sweet potato
- ✓ Food made with whole grains and no added sugar

Worst Choices

- ✗ Processed grains, such as white rice or white flour
- ✗ Cereals loaded with sugar
- ✗ White bread
- ✗ French fries

Fiber

Fiber is not absorbed into the bloodstream like other foods, but it is an essential nutrient. Eating fiber-rich foods like vegetables and fruits will provide you with a feeling of satiety. Being full will eventually help you in regulating your appetite and controlling your blood sugar.

Fiber also lubricates the stomach and intestinal lining preventing constipation. Nuts, legumes, whole-wheat flour are some of the foods you can and should incorporate into your diet.

Best Choices

- ✓ Fresh veggies or eaten raw, lightly steamed, grilled or boiled.
- ✓ Greens such as arugula, spinach, and kale.

Worst Choices

- ✗ Canned vegetables because of their sodium content
- ✗ Veggies cooked with butter, sauce, cheese.
- ✗ Pickles and sauerkraut

Fish

While the temptation of indulging in a well-made steak is great, you need to control your cravings. Red meat and diabetes do not mix. What you need to do is find alternatives and fish is a great option. It is not only heat-friendly but also very rich in nutrients.

Make a point of eating white meat, mainly fish at least twice a week. There are great examples that you can choose from; tuna, sardines (very rich in Omega-3 fatty acids), codfish, salmon, mackerel, halibut, sea bass, pompano, herring, lake trout, and bluefish. Since they are rich in omega-3 fatty acids, they are known to be heart friendly and have lower levels of triglycerides and cholesterol to circulate in your bloodstream. But remember, As much as fish is healthy, fried fish is dangerous to your health.

Polyunsaturated fats

Examples of vegetable oils under the category of polyunsaturated fats are corn, soybean, safflower, sunflower and cottonseed oils. These polyunsaturated fats are a good substitute for saturated and trans fats that help to improve your good HDL over your bad LDL cholesterol.

Monounsaturated fats

Monounsaturated fats are the same with polyunsaturated fats as they remain liquid at room temperature in your grocery shelves. The example of vegetable oils under this category are olive oil, canola oil, avocados and peanut oil.

These help to lower your bad cholesterol without affecting the LDL good cholesterol.

What not to eat

Not all fats are good for your body. In your journey of controlling diabetes naturally through diet, you need to make a point of staying clear of:

Saturated Fats

Saturated fats are notorious for raising the levels of cholesterol in your body. High cholesterol in your body is not only a risk factor for diabetes, but also for your heart.

Lad, cream sauces, butter, high-fat milk, salt pork, poultry skin, meat puddings are some of the foods that are high in saturated fats.

Trans fats

The trans fats also increase the level of blood cholesterol in the body. It is more dangerous than the saturated fats. Trans fats are made when liquid oil solidifies under room temperature (hydrogenation). Sources of the fat include shortening, margarine, processed foods, and baked goods.

It is a good ideal for you to read the food label labels of every product you buy to see how much saturated fat it contains.

Cholesterol

The body makes a substantial amount of cholesterol, but the rest comes from the diets that you choose. Overeating cholesterol will increase its levels in the body. It is advisable to take < 300 mg per day. Foods rich in cholesterol include poultry skin, liver, egg yolks, and high-fat dairy products.

Sodium

High levels of sodium in the blood increase the risk of hypertension. But, you should not eliminate sodium from your diet completely as you need. Lower and intake of about < 2,300 mg per day.

You also need to avoid the following foods that are high in sugar, carbs and calorie content.

Coffee Drinks

Coffee drinks that you purchased from the coffee-shops contain high calorie, carb, and fat contents. They usually contain whole milk, lots of sugar, syrup, high-fat creamer etc.

Soft drinks, Fruit Juice Beverages and Flavored Water

Everybody's favorite, these beverages are some of the worst foods for diabetes as they are all very high in sugar content and calories. For every can of soda, there is 33g of sugar. For a cup of fruit juice, there is 23g of sugar. For every can of flavored water, there is 6g of sugar. You wouldn't want these sugars to worsen your diabetes, right?

Cookies, Cakes, and Doughnuts

Cookies, cakes, and doughnuts contain a high amount of trans fats, sugars, and carbs. Their ingredients contain some of the worst saturated fats and trans fats which are butter, high-fructose corn syrup, margarine, butter, shortening and partially hydrogenated and pure hydrogenated oils. They also contain granulated sugar, maple syrup, sucralose, molasses and much more which pile up even more on the calorie and carb content.

Processed Foods and Canned Goods

Packaged and processed foods are affordable and convenient to eat. Some of these are hot dogs, hams, corned beef, and sausages, just to name a few. However, these contain lots of fats, sodium, and sugar. Living with diabetes should take these foods off your shopping list. If this becomes a habit, it is now time to break it by not relying on these whenever you get hungry. It may be a quick meal, but It is never a safe bet. To start eating healthy, you should be able to plan ahead before going to the grocery.

Deep-Fried Chinese Entrees

So you've just stepped out of your house to go on an errand, and suddenly you start thinking about your favorite Chinese restaurant. Unfortunately, this is not a smart food choice. While some dishes might be a great choice, you might as well pass on items which are deep fried like fried orange chicken and steamed white rice. Stop and think about it for a minute, the chicken has already breaded in white flour, deep fried in a cooking oil and dipped in a sauce already has more than 400 calories, 50 grams of carbohydrates per serving. Now, since you are going to eat it with steamed with white rice, there will be another 200 calories and 45 grams of carbohydrates from this in a usual 1-cup serving. Getting the extra rice would add more. Moreover, it also does not contain any vegetable.

Controlling Diabetes Naturally Through Exercise

Exercise contributes around 20% to your weight management goal. There are of course a variety of exercises available. However, as a person with diabetes, you need to focus on the exercises that will help you to lose weight and give you energy.

Before you start exercising, it is crucial for you to consult your doctor on the proper exercise routines for you. You also need to ensure that you monitor your blood sugar before and after exercising. It is **important** for you to exercise in favorable weather conditions. You don't want to be caught outside exercising in bad weather.

The main goal of exercise is to: improve insulin resistance, improve the lipid profile (lowering the cholesterol), maintain the ideal body weight, and lifestyle.

Great Exercises

Walking

Walking is fun and effective, but it should be done as directed by your doctor. Most doctors recommend brisk walking that can raise your heartbeat. It is advisable for you to take a nice walk at least three times a week. Many doctors also advise you to do aerobics exercises when possible. Walking is a simple low-stress exercise routine, but it should be done properly and when I say this I mean the right gear. Probably one of the best investment you can make for this particular exercise is a good pair of running or walking shoes.

Before you start walking, it is essential for you to warm-up and check your breathing rate. Start off slowly and build on your speed as you go. You can also incorporate other workout techniques as you go. If you experience shortness of breath, stop the exercise and wait a few minutes before continuing.

Yoga and dancing

Yoga is an accepted form of exercise because of its many benefits. Yoga helps in improving your general mood and your nerve functions, as well as limber up your body. The exercise also helps in improving your muscle mass which in turn helps to lower your blood sugar. Engaging in yoga sessions once or twice a week will help improve your mental health.

Dancing is a great workout routine. It is an all-rounded exercise as it works on all your body muscles as well as improve your heart rate. It doesn't matter if you don't know how to dance the idea is to move your body. You can join a Zumba class to help you in your moves.

Swimming

Swimming helps you to burn body fat faster than many other workout routines. As you begin swimming you may have huge expectations that may be unrealistic. Working out in the pool is different from other exercises. Swimming requires a combination of both your muscles and cardiovascular system. Your lungs also need to adjust to the change in environment. For that reason, you need to swim in measured segments or intervals.

Incorporating other swimming techniques will also help you attain your goal. As you swim, you need to exercise caution to avoid cuts. Open wounds and cuts heal slowly due to your reduced immune system and can also increase the risk of infections. There are even special shoes that are designed to be used in the pool.

Tai Chi

For centuries, the Tai Chi has been used to reduce stress and anxiety. Due to the many benefits, the exercise routines are suitable for diabetic patients across the globe. The exercises include slow and controlled movements in intervals of 30 minutes. Tai Chi helps in enhancing balance and flexibility and general mood. It also helps in lowering blood pressure.

If you can't engage in Tai Chi, you need to choose other balance related exercise to help you in your flexibility.

Weight training

Weight training is not only for diabetic patients but also for all persons as well. The exercises help in building the muscle mass which is crucial for the diabetic patients. Loss of muscle mass leads to the inability to control the blood sugar. You should try to schedule a weight training exercise at least twice a week.

Cycling

Cycling, just like swimming is an all-rounded exercise. The exercises help in increasing the cardiovascular fitness and muscle strength. It also helps to strengthen your bones, improve your posture, and joint mobility. With cycling, you can reduce your overall body fat levels.

You can also opt for stationary exercise bikes as they have the same effect as writing a real bike on your body.

Tips for working out

- ✓ It is vital for you to have a workout partner to help keep you motivated. Joining a workout group or a gym can be a great way to exercise.
- ✓ You to set your workout goals before you begin. Having actionable goals will help you take note of your progress.
- ✓ Be sure to hydrate by drinking lots of water.

- ✓ Have a fruit juice, sports drink or a snack on you at all times in case hypoglycemia occurs.
- ✓ Don't overdo it, and always call for help if you are in pain

Managing Through Medication

The doctor may prescribe certain medicines based on the type of diabetes and the severity of your case.

Insulin

The drug is usually given to persons with diabetic type 1. However, the doctor may still recommend it for people with diabetes type 2. There are various options available:

- ✓ The short-acting insulin:
- ✓ Rapid-acting insulin
- ✓ Long-acting insulin
- ✓ Intermediate-acting insulin
- ✓ Combination insulin

Insulin medication is given to replace the insulin not being produced by your body.

Amylinomimetic Drug

The drug is given as an injection, and it is administered before meals. It helps in the reduction of glucagon production which happens after meals. The drug also helps in reducing the appetite and giving a sense of satiety (it slows down digestion and the absorption of food).

Alpha-glucosidase inhibitors

The drugs help in the breakdown of sugar and starchy foods and thus lowering the blood sugar. The drugs are taken before meals for better results. They include miglitol and acarbose.

Biguanides

These drugs (Kazano, Invokamet, Synjardy, Glucovance) are designed to decrease the amount of sugar that the intestines can absorb. This will make your body sensitive to the insulin produced. The drugs also help in decreasing the amount of sugar that the liver can make.

DPP-4 inhibitors

The drugs are responsible for promoting the production of insulin in the body. They help in the reduction of blood sugar levels but also protect the body from hypoglycemia. The drugs include the Nesina, Kazano, Oseni, Glyxambi, and Onglyza among others.

Glucagon-peptides

These drugs help is the promotion of B-cell growth. They also help in determining how much insulin the body can produce at any given time. The significantly reduce your appetite. Drugs like Tanzeum, Byetta, Bydureon, and Victoza fall under this category.

SGLT 2 Inhibitors (Sodium-glucose transporter)

The drugs help in the prevention of glucose hold-up in the kidneys. The excess glucose in the body is excreted through urine. The drugs include the Farxiga, Invokana, Jardiance, Xigduo XR, Invokamet, Glyxambi, and Synjardy.

Meglitinides

They promote the release of the insulin. One of the associated side effects is the drugs can cause hypoglycemia. Because of that, they are not designed for everyone, and you should consult a doctor before taking the medication. The drugs in this category include the Nateglinide, Prandimet, and Repaglinide.

Sulfonylureas

These drugs help stimulate the pancreas promoting the production of insulin. The drugs in this category include the Amaryl, Duetact, Avandaryl, Metaglip, Gliclazide, Glucotrol, Tolinase, and Diabinese among others.

Thiazolidinediones

The drugs help in decreasing of the glucose level in the liver. They also encourage fat cells to utilize the already secreted insulin. The side effect of the drugs is the increased risk of heart disease. The drugs include Actos, Oseni, Avandia, and Duetact.

Diabetic patients also take other medication to help reduce the associated complications. They can take drugs to control high cholesterol levels and high blood pressure.

Exercises and medication are essential for you. However, diabetes can't be managed without paying attention to the diet. Your diet will determine how successful you will be in managing the condition. It is important that you consult a registered dietician to help you in designing a suitable diet plan to help you control your diabetes. It is crucial for you to control your portions and your calorie intake.

Chapter 4:

Why Managing Diabetes Naturally is Preferred

Diabetes has no cure, and that is the sad truth that we all have to face. However, with the proper information, you can manage the condition and lead a happy lifestyle. Diabetes, for many years, has been controlled with insulin shots and that is what most people know as the remedy. But, did you know that insulin is not the only way that you can regulate your blood sugar? Yes, it is totally possible for you to live without the painful injections.

Alternative therapies are available today and can be used to control the disease. Considering the natural remedies may be risky, especially if you have been using the insulin shots for a long period of time. However, the benefits of using the natural remedies far outweigh the cons.

Why you should consider the natural remedies

Prescription drugs come with their own set of problems. Yes, they will help you in regulating your blood sugar, but some of them may have adverse side effects. There are those medications that significantly lower your blood glucose causing hypoglycemia. Some of them due to their chemical makeup can even put you at risk of heart disease.

Diabetes is a disease that doesn't exist alone. It is often associated with other complications. To achieve optimal health, you may need to take other drugs to deal with these associated conditions. Taking too many medications will have a toll on your already compromised immunity. The result could be an increased risk of infections.

What about the financial aspect? The insulin and diabetic medications are not cheap, and if you don't have insurance, you may have to pay for the necessary medications to control your diabetes out-of-pocket.

Using the natural remedies will help you eliminate some if not all of the side effects caused by prescription diabetes medications. The treatments especially herbal supplements have natural ingredients that will help you not only in the regulation of your blood sugar but also in improving your general health. The herbal supplements are relatively cheap and readily available in most pharmacies.

The Alternative Therapies

Considerable research has been performed in the use of alternative remedies that diabetic patients can adapt. While a lot more needs to be done, the information that is already available is promising.

Physical intervention

It is not about treating diabetes with medication only, physical therapies can go a long way in ensuring you maintain healthy blood sugar levels in your body as well.

Yoga

For years, Yoga has been used to promote relaxation and improving the general mood. Yoga helps in controlling the symptoms associated with type 2 diabetes. A yoga routine also helps in managing the complications that come with the disease. Yoga helps those with diabetes to regulate their body functions. Also, with a regular Yoga routine, you can enjoy increased flexibility, respiration function, and vitality. The exercise also helps to improve your muscle strength which is vital for you to maintain healthy blood glucose levels.

Acupuncture

Acupuncture is mostly used in China as a pain alleviating therapy. In the last few decades, the treatment has begun to see use in some diabetic patients as well. The treatment has been beneficial in the management of diabetes and also in the control of the associated diabetic complications.

Clinical research done on animals has indicated that acupuncture can promote the glucose-6-phosphate. The treatment can also stimulate the pancreas and eventually increase the production of insulin. It also helps in the utilization of the blood glucose, lowering the level of sugar in the bloodstream.

Massage therapy

Even though massage therapy is used for relaxation purposes, it is quite beneficial to diabetic patients. Massage therapy can help in reducing the heart rate and regulating blood pressure. It helps in improving blood circulation in the body which will, in turn, improving nerve function and help to alleviate pain. Massage therapy stimulates your lymph system and also increase insulin sensitivity in the body. This is achieved through the control of some stress hormones.

Before you consider beginning a massage therapy, it is crucial for you to consult your doctors on the safe way to proceed.

The herbal medicines

Neem

Neem is ranked as one of the safest natural herb supplements. The production of the supplement is done naturally, and thus there is no human interference. Due to this, the herb presents small or no side effects. The herb is extracted from the leaves of the neem plant.

This herbal supplement helps in lowering the blood sugar in the body. It helps to prevent the glucose-induced hyperglycemia and also prevents the production of adrenaline.

Neem leaves contain flavonoid, anti-viral compounds, triterpenoid, and glycosides. These compounds help in lowering the glucose in the bloodstream. The compounds block the epinephrine in the body thus promoting glucose utilization in the body.

Bitter melon

Bitter melon is not only fruit but also an herbal medicine. It contains ingredients that are beneficial to diabetic patients. The fruit has Charatin (helps in lowering the blood levels), polypeptide-p (insulin-like compounds), and Vicine.

Lectin is another active ingredient in the fruit. It acts on the peripheral tissue and thus lowers the blood glucose. Lectin also helps in suppressing appetite.

Fenugreek

It is a common ingredient in most Indian cuisine because of its strong aromatic flavor. Despite being an active ingredient in many recipes, the herb has great benefits on diabetes.

The seeds are high in fiber which helps to slow down digestion and thus reducing the blood sugar. The herb has also been linked to the lowering of the of the lipid levels in the body.

Fenugreek is rich in vitamins and also minerals which help to improve your overall health. Due to its ingredients, the herb can be used to treat some of the kidney ailments and the ED caused by diabetes.

Cinnamon

It is an aromatic herb/ spice that is extracted from the bark of the cinnamon trees. The spice is mostly used in cooking, but it is also used as an herbal supplement in the treatment of diabetes.

The spice imitates insulin in the body thus increasing the glucose sensitivity in the body. The spice also helps in lowering the blood sugar level by increasing the insulin sensitivity.

Oxidative stress has been linked to increasing the onset of diabetes. Taking cinnamon supplements will reduce the oxidative stress that causes cell damage. Antioxidants are active ingredients in the spice which help in fighting the free radicals.

Cinnamon plays a vital role in the fasting glucose and the post-meals blood sugar. In both cases, it helps to lower the blood sugar. It helps to regulate the digestion thus reducing the rate the stomach empties itself.

There are two types of cinnamon spices; the Ceylon and Cassia. The two are distinct when it comes to their properties. Cassia comes from a combination of cinnamon trees. It is readily available and is inexpensive. You will find it in most food stores were pharmacies in the vitamin section. The Ceylon is extracted from the Cinnamon Verum. It is rich in antioxidants and thus very expensive. Due to the extraction process of the spice, Ceylon is not as easily available.

Cassia cinnamon is lower in antioxidants. It can also be harmful to some people as it contains Coumarin. The ingredient can lead to liver toxicity. The spice should be taken in moderation and according to the direction of a doctor.

Grapeseed Extract

Grape seed extract is rich in natural ingredients. The seeds contain the Pycnogenol, an antioxidant that benefits the cardiovascular system greatly. It helps in lowering the inflammation of in the blood vessels and improving the blood viscosity.

It also helps to improve the microcirculation which will lower your blood sugar levels. Not only does it reduce the sugar levels in the bloodstream, but it also helps to speed up the healing process. Most diabetic patients have a compromised immunity which affects their healing power. The supplement significantly increased the healing process among the diabetic patients with leg ulcers (causes leg amputation)

Grape seed extract helped to improve the abnormalities found in the small blood vessels. It also leads to the decrease of capillary function and lowered symptoms of edema.

The Pycnogenol helps to reduce the progression of the eye infections in people with diabetes.

Grape seed extracts also help in the management of associated diabetic complications. With its antioxidants, the extract lowers the risk of heart disease. The seeds contain anti-inflammatory properties that promote blood flow. They also help to prevent thickening of the blood.

Mango leaves

Mango leaves contain compounds like caffeinic acid, Mangiferin, flavonoids, and gallic which help in the regulation of the blood glucose.

The leaves, through the caffeinic acid, help to lower the body's blood sugar levels. They also promote the distribution and utilization of the glucose in the blood.

The mango leaves are rich in pectin which helps in lowering the cholesterol levels. They are also rich in Vitamin C (improves the immune function) and fiber which aids in better food digestion.

Mango leaves contain Vitamin A which is linked to better vision. The supplement also helps in delaying the progression of retinopathy.

To use the leaves, you need to boil them and allow the liquid to cool overnight before you drink it. For effective results, drink the water before meals.

Vitamin C

This essential vitamin is found in oranges, mangoes, pineapples, guava, papaya (it is rich in antioxidants), and spinach among others. Vitamin C helps in lowering the blood sugar levels to within normal levels. The Vitamin also helps to improve your compromised immunity.

Aloe Vera

Aloe Vera is curative. It is not only beneficial to your skin and hair, but also in lowering the lipid levels in the body. The plant helps in accelerating the healing process of ulcers and wounds.

Herbal supplements are great not only for the management of diabetes but also for your general health. However, as a diabetic patient, you need to proceed with caution when you are taking the herbs. It is vital to consult a doctor on the types of herbal supplements that you can safely use.

Dietary supplements

Vitamins and minerals play a vital role in the normal functioning of the body. The vitamins and minerals function as co-factors for body metabolic reactions. If you have diabetes, it is important for you to take the supplements to help promote proper body functions.

Chromium

Chromium is a trace element. It is essential for normal glucose metabolism maintenance. The minerals functions as a coenzyme for the insulin activities in the body. Due to that, the mineral is a determinant for the sensitivity of insulin in the body. Without the mineral, the insulin action will be blocked, and you will experience elevated blood glucose.

Chromium promotes the uptake of glucose in the body and also facilitates the binding of insulin. Taking the supplements will help in improving glucose tolerance and decreasing the fasting blood sugar level. It also helps to decrease the levels of cholesterol in the body and also lower the levels of insulin.

Taking chromium supplements is recommended, but it should be done under the supervision of the doctor. A high dose of the mineral can lead to hypoglycemia.

Magnesium

Magnesium deficiency is common among persons with diabetes. Low levels of magnesium have been linked to increased levels of diabetes. Having low levels of magnesium will increase your risk to diabetic complications like retinopathy. It is important to take a magnesium supplement as dietary magnesium is insufficient in the body.

Vanadium

Vanadium exists in its natural form and has not yet been categorized as an essential nutrient. Research has indicated that the mineral is beneficial to persons with diabetes type 1. However, the persons with diabetes mellitus can also benefit from the supplement as it helps in increasing the sensitivity of insulin in the body.

Vitamin E

Vitamin E is a fat-soluble vitamin that acts as an antioxidant in the body. Low levels of the vitamin have been linked to increased risk of diabetes.

Hyperglycemia leads to the increased levels of free radicals. For that reason, persons with diabetes require higher levels of antioxidants. Vitamin E supplement will decrease the levels of oxidative stress produced by free radicals.

The above-mentioned natural therapies can be beneficial no doubt. But, before you use any of them, be sure to consult with your doctor in order to avoid any possible complications.

Chapter 5:

Choosing a Diet to Help You Control Your Diabetes

Food is everywhere you look, and it can be tempting to eat the foods that you see. However, when you have diabetes, you can't just eat what you want and expect to manage your blood sugar successfully. Yes, some people bow down to their cravings, but that can be harmful to your blood sugar and overall health. Paying attention to what you feed your body is your ticket to a healthier lifestyle.

Did you know that your habits influence your food selection? You subconsciously choose what to eat at any given time. Your habits affect what you eat when you eat, where you eat, and even who you eat with.

If you hope to succeed in regulating your blood sugar levels, you need to be aware of your eating habits and how they are formed.

You don't just sit around and come up with your personal food preferences; they are formed and determined by several factors.

Some of the eating habits

Eating while hungry

Ever heard of the saying 'never go to the grocery store when you are hungry,' well this should be applied to eating too. Hunger is a cue for eating food. However, most people when they feel hunger, tend to reach out for carbohydrates since they are one of the energy giving foods. Eating when you feel hungry will lead to overeating. If you have diabetes, you can't afford to have hyperglycemia immediately after eating. To avoid this, you need to learn about portion control. It is advised for you to eat small portions of food at least four times a day, instead of eating a giant plate of food at once.

Judging the food by taste

Taste of food is influenced by different experiences in our lives. Most people lean more towards the sweet foods than the sour or bland ones. Yes, you should focus on the taste of the food. But, focusing on the 'sweet' foods can be costly. If you don't like the taste of the healthy foods, there are various ways that you can improve it. Think twice before you eat that candy bar next time!

Buying the food based on the price tag

Living healthy can be expensive. You should try to buy wholemeal foods and grains to meet your health needs. The cost of the food is a factor that influences your habits. It is not necessary for you to break the bank to live a healthy life, you can find cheaper alternatives that can meet your daily nutrient requirements.

Some rich people buy food based on the price tag. Did you know that there are foods created for the affluent? Yes, food like fried chicken, burgers, pizzas, and sodas that cater to the wealthy. The fact that the food item is expensive doesn't mean it is nutrient-rich. Take your time to read the food labels before you buy the food.

Eating with your emotions

Hunger is not the only reason why people eat food. There are many people who have formed the habit of eating while they are stressed or sad. While it is perfectly fine to find a stress reliever, food should not be an option. Unfortunately, food, unlike other forms of relieving stress like working out, will affect your body and general health negatively.

Eating while watching television

Most people tend to eat when they are watching football or a movie which is fine. The problem with this habit is the choice of food you choose. Pay attention to what you choose to eat, and you won't have to worry about shedding those extra pounds.

Conforming to the social convention

When you attend a party, at times, you don't have control over what will be served. But, if you are diabetic, you can't afford to eat just anything. You can either inform the host about your diet choices, or better still bring your own food.

Sleep eating

Sleep eating is a severe eating disorder that is characterized with compulsive eating and drinking while asleep. Sleep eating occurs even when the feelings of hunger are absent. Binge eating can result in serious health issues. It is important for you to talk to a doctor about the issue. Identifying your trigger can also help you in regulating the issue. But, as you wait for your brain to adjust to the medication, you can choose to fill your pantry with healthy food. It might not be a lasting solution, but it will keep you from binging on unhealthy foods.

Not paying attention to what you eat

It goes without saying that nutrition knowledge is power. Lack of nutrition information will lead to a poor diet. It is vital for you to spend some time reading about the foods that you need to be eating. Reading on diabetes and how to manage it will help learn how to maintain the blood sugar levels with proper nutrition.

Rushing through time

Working people find it hard to cook at home due to the time constraints and thus they mostly eat out. No rule exists that it is mandatory to eat a home-cooked meal. However, when you are trying to manage your diabetes, you need to be cautious about the foods that you order in restaurants.

Improving your diets

Improving your eating habits will make it easy to manage a diabetic diet. There are a few tips that you should consider. Use the three Rs; Reflect, replace, and reinforce.

- ✓ Keep a list of your food intake for a few days. Make a point of writing down everything that you eat during these days and also the time of day that you eat it.
- ✓ Take an inventory of your unhealthy eating habits.
- ✓ Identify all your triggers. Take note of the times you eat for reasons other than hunger. Some of the triggers can be moods, stress, idling, and cravings
- ✓ If you are an emotional eater, talk to a counselor on how to thoroughly to manage your emotions
- ✓ Replace the unhealthy foods with healthy ones
- ✓ Reinforce the diet that you have adapted
- ✓ Be patient as forming new habits can take time.

Factors to consider when choosing a diet

When it comes to choosing your diets, you need to be actively involved in the process. The primary goals of planning your meal are to:

- ✓ Lower your blood sugar
- ✓ Lower your blood cholesterol
- ✓ Improve your muscle mass
- ✓ Improve your immunity

- ✓ Provide you with energy
- ✓ Improve your general mood

You need to, therefore, choose diets that will bring you closer to your overall goals.

Dietary requirements for managing diabetes naturally

Meeting your nutritional requirement is crucial in lowering your blood glucose. Only a balanced diet can help you meet your daily needs. Your daily diet should include vegetables, fruits, proteins, and plenty of whole grains.

It is important for you to learn about these foods to help you in proper dietary planning. The foundation of every meal should be plant-based foods when possible.

The nutrients of every food group differ. Combining different foods in a single meal will promote proper nutrition. Adding other ingredients and spices will not only improve the quality of the food but will also improve your general health.

The portion sizes of the foods are essential. Your dietician can tell you what size the portions need to be in order to maintain a healthy nutritional balance in every meal. When you are buying the foods in a food store, take time to read the labels for guidelines of the portions.

The different portion sizes of foods

- A serving of fish is equivalent to 3 ounces
- A serving of whole grains is equal to ½ cup of cereals, one slice of bread, ½ cup of sweet potatoes
- A serving of fruits is equivalent to ½ one cup of diced fruit
- A serving of dairy milk (non-fat) is one cup

You need to pay attention to the intake of sugar and sodium. You don't need processed sugar, you can get your daily intake of sugar from a variety of sources including honey and fruits. When it comes to sodium, you should not eliminate it from your diet. You can only limit the intake to the required daily allowance which is about 2300mg per day.

Incorporate healthy fats into your daily diet. Salmon, avocados, nuts, peanuts, and tuna are sources of healthy 'fats.

Pay attention to your age group when it comes to planning your diet. For example, persons above the age of 50 years need more calcium than young adults, and older adults require more Vitamin A.

Allergies

Do you have any food allergies that must be considered? Are you a vegetarian? These are some of the questions that you will need to consider when you are choosing your diet.

A diabetic diet is already restricted when it comes to the types of foods. If you are vegetarian, you will need to add more options in your diet to meet your daily requirement.

Do you have any existing health problems that require special diets? If you have any of the associated diabetic complications, you need to plan your diet to address the issues.

Religion

Religion plays a significant role in the type of foods that you can eat. If your religion prohibits you from taking certain foods, you need to discuss this with the dietician to find healthy alternatives.

The cost of the food

As mentioned above, the prices of food influence your choice of food and will affect your diet. Planning your meals will benefit you greatly. Make a list of all the foods that you need to buy in advance before you go shopping.

Your activity level

There are two types of diabetic patients active and moderately active persons. Your activity level will influence your diet. If you are active, you need a more nutrient-rich and also high-calorie diet to help meet your energy requirement.

Consider the benefits and side effects

Every diet offers a different set of benefits to you. However, not all great diets that you come across are designed for you. You need to take your time to do research on the different types of diet plans available (if you don't want to design yourself). Learn about their effectiveness and side effects that they might have.

Preferences

Your personal preference will play a vital role in the type of diet and food that you choose. The fact that you are eating healthy doesn't mean you should eat foods that you don't like. Your preference here doesn't refer to choosing pizza over a bowl of salad. It means choosing to eat spinach instead of broccoli, or eating a mango instead of a pineapple etc.

Choosing your food is one thing, and planning the meal is another. Certain methods can be used to help you in preparing your meals.

Plate method

It is the simplest method for ensuring you plan your meals efficiently. With this plan, you need to have ½ a plate of non-starchy vegetables (choose a variety), ¼ of protein (fish and skinless chicken), and ¼ of starch (whole grains).

Food pyramid

The pyramid organizes the food in seven tiers including starch, milk, fruits, vegetables, meat, fats, and sugars.

Food exchange system

Food comes in six categories; starch (grains, cereals, pasta, starchy vegetables, and beans), meat and its substitutes, fruits, milk, non-starchy vegetables, and fats. With the help of a dietician, you can plan your meals based on the serving requirements of these food categories. The system will allow you to measure your serving portions easily. It will save you time as any food can be substituted for another as long as they belong to the same category.

Types of diets to choose from

You have several options that you can choose from when it comes to diet. Before you can plan your meals, it is important to note that it's not about eating healthy, but also the timing.

If you notice your blood sugar level is low before bedtime, you should take slow carbohydrates (they are digested and absorbed slowly). It will prevent hypoglycemia at night headaches, night sweats, and restless sleep. Night time hypoglycemia will lead to elevated blood sugar by morning.

Even though you may be hyperglycemic when you wake up, you should never skip your breakfast. There are few healthy options that you can choose. Skipping breakfast is detrimental to your general health, and it may also lower your insulin sensitivity.

G.I Diets

They are referred to as glycemic index diets that are designed based on the level of carbohydrates in the food. Doctors and dieticians use the G.I index list to plan the meals. The G.I determines how a portion of food will raise your blood sugar level after you consume it. The diets are based on carbohydrates containing foods that are less likely to increase your blood sugar.

People use the diets to;

- ✓ Lose or maintain their weight
- ✓ To manage their blood sugar
- ✓ To improve their general health
- ✓ Increase the body's insulin sensitivity

The G.I values are divided into three;

- Low G.I foods (1 to 55): they are digested and absorbed slowly. The meals include non-starchy vegetables, fruits, pasta, oatmeal, whole wheat, sweet potato, yam, corn, legumes, lentils, butter beans, and carrots.
- Medium G.I (56 to 69): the foods include whole wheat, pita bread, rye, brown or basmati rice, and quick oats.
- High G.I (70 or higher): the foods include white bread, corn flakes, short grain rice, macaroni and cheese, rice cakes, popcorn, pineapple, and rice pasta.

The glycemic index is affected by different factors like the fat and fiber content in the food. Cooking methods can also increase the overall G.I of the food. Other factors include; processing food (orange juice has a higher GI than eating whole fruit), ripeness and storage of the foods, and variety (brown rice has a higher GI compared to the long-grain white rice).

Principles of Glycemic Diet Plan

Eat more fiber

Fiber helps by slowing down the digestion of food thereby stabilizing your blood sugar. Avoid refined foods when possible because the more processed the food is, the less fiber it will contain.

Eat your carbohydrates in their original state

Processed foods tend to have a higher glycemic index and load.

Combine carbohydrates with proteins

Combining different low GI foods is essential as it will help in the management of your glucose level.

Pritikin diets

Pritikin diets are low in fat and high in fiber. The food in this type of diet include fruits, vegetables, potatoes, yams, corn, non-fat dairy products, whole bread, oatmeal, brown rice, non-fat yogurt, fish, fortified soy milk, skinless chicken, soybeans, tofu, and legumes.

With the Pritikin diets, you need to avoid the saturated fats (coconut, cheese, whole milk, and butter), organ meats, bacon, hot dogs, bologna, vegetable oils, and egg yolks.

The Pritikin diets are fine when it comes to regulating the blood sugar. However, they should be taken in combination with exercises to avoid any possible diabetic complications.

Here are some simple tips that will help you with the Pritikin diet;

- ✓ Start any meal with a salad, fruit, soup or whole grain. These foods will help you to fill up before the main dish limiting the possibility of eating high-calorie meals.
- ✓ Avoid taking high-calorie drinks like soda. Taking a glass of wine is great for your heart, but you should avoid drinking alcoholic drinks.
- ✓ Eat a healthy snack in between the meals. They will give you energy and limit the chances of overeating.
- ✓ Eat lots of fish like salmon and codfish.
- ✓ Quit smoking if you are a smoker.

Vegan Diets

Vegan diets that are low in saturated fat and cholesterol and can help you regulate your blood glucose levels. You should ensure that every meal is rich in protein and fiber. A vegan diet refers to cutting down on the dairy, meat, and other animal products.

The foods that you should eat are vegetables, grains, legumes, and fruits. Starting your vegan diet will be hard and will require a lot of compromise and adjustment on your part. However, investing your time to understand how to balance the foods will make it easy for you to adjust.

When you are taking the vegan diet, you may need to take vitamin B12 supplements.

Varieties of Vegan Diets

The raw vegan diet

It is based on consuming raw vegetables, fruits, and nuts

The whole food diet

The diet is comprised of whole foods like fruits, vegetables, legumes, whole grains, and nuts

Low-fat vegan diet

With this diet, you limit the intake of food rich in fat like avocados and nuts.

Vegan diets can be limiting when it comes to the nutrients and may lead to severe nutrient deficiency. So, before you can start a vegan diet, it is important for you to consult your doctor on the right way to proceed.

Vegan diets promote weight loss. But, they also lower your blood sugar and increase insulin sensitivity in the body.

Paleo diets

The purpose of Paleo diet is to eat like the cavemen did in the stone-age era. The diet promotes weight loss. With this diet, you should eat eggs, seeds, nuts, and the healthy oils. On the other hand, you should avoid refined sugar, dairy products, refined vegetable oil, potatoes, and salt.

You won't have to count the calories with this diet. The Paleo diet is rich in fiber as it involves eating a lot of fruits and vegetables.

The diet presents you with both pros and cons;

Pros

- ✓ The diet focuses on unprocessed and whole foods. You fill up on fruits and whole vegetables.
- ✓ You will eat less simple carbohydrates. Carbohydrates are best-eaten whole. Simple carbohydrates lead to elevated blood sugar as they are easily digested and contain a high GI. With paleo diets, you will avoid the consumption of the refined and processed carbohydrates.

Cons

- ✗ Paleo diets are restrictive. The diet forbids the intake of foods that are rich in essential nutrients. Most paleo diets recommend eliminating legumes, dairy and dairy-derived products.
- ✗ Costly: eating fish and white meat can substantially raise your grocery bill
- ✗ There is not a lot of information available on paleo diets.

If you want to follow this diet, you need focus on eating food rich in proteins and the healthy fats.

Keep in mind that paleo diet is a low-carb diet and thus it may lead to hypoglycemia. You need to proceed with caution, and as always consider consulting your doctor before you begin.

Low-carb diets

Low-carb diets have allowed the people living with diabetes mellitus to normalize their blood sugar level.

Carbohydrate has the most significant effect on your blood sugar. But, the nutrients are essential for your body as they provide energy. Instead of eliminating carbohydrates (which will prove difficult to do), you are advised to lower your carbs intake instead.

Benefits of using the low-carb diet

- ✓ weight loss
- ✓ lower HbA1c
- ✓ increased energy levels
- ✓ lower risk of diabetic complications
- ✓ improved mind activity
- ✓ fewer cravings
- ✓ decreased risk of hyperglycemia.

A low-carb diet allows you to choose the level of carbohydrates that are suitable for your condition. Low carbohydrates mean an intake of carbs that are under 130g of carbohydrates.

The lower the level of carb intake, the lower your blood sugar level will be.

What a healthy low-carb diet should have

- ✓ Moderate intake of protein
- ✓ Low or limited consumption of processed food, grains, and sugar
- ✓ Intake of fat from natural sources: like avocado, nuts, olive oil, eggs, fish, and olives.
- ✓ Increased intake of whole vegetables

If you reduce the consumption of carbohydrates, you need to increase the intake of protein or fatty foods to make up for the reduced number of calories.

The low-carb diet is associated with constipation, fatigue, headaches, decreased concentration, and some nutrient deficiencies.

Tips for making the meal tasty

The fact that you have to eat healthily it doesn't mean that the food should be boring and blunt. It is easy to modify the recipes and make them friendly.

Replace the solid fats with liquid oils

As a person with diabetes, you should avoid saturated fats and the Trans fats. If the recipe that you choose calls for butter or any other form of solid fat, you can replace them with trans-fat-free oils like margarine, and spreads. Olive oil, corn oil, and grape seed oil can work perfectly in some of the recipes.

Replace the high-fat dairy

Most of the baking and cooking recipes use the high-fat dairy products which are not allowed in diabetic diets. You can use the low-diary fats, and lower the fat content in the food without changing the taste of the food. For example, if the food recipe that you choose calls for whole milk, you can choose non-fat half and a half or skim milk.

Experiment with flavors

Adding spices to your meal can make all the difference. Make use of spices like cinnamon, cardamom, mustard, nutmeg, basil, and a mix of herbs. These spices are also great for your general health.

No diet is similar to the other. Some are good, and different diets are limiting. When it comes to planning your diets, you need to choose a diet that will work for your body.

Chapter 6:

Diets in Detail

Dieticians say 'a minute on the mouth is a lifetime on the hips.' It may appear as a cliché, but it's true. You can't just eat what you want all the time and expect to live a healthy lifestyle. If you want to see or even fulfill your lifetime dreams, you have to start eating healthy and began exercising regularly. That is the only proven technique of living a long, fulfilling life.

Dieticians and scientists alike have developed a variety of diets that can enable you to stay healthy and strong. Most of the diets offer great benefits to your body, but one size doesn't always fit all. You will need to talk to a doctor or a registered dietician for guidance on designing a suitable diet for your needs.

The types of diets

Mediterranean diets

Mediterranean diets are heart-friendly. The diets are based on foods cooked in the Mediterranean style. The meals will comprise of basic foods with a sprinkle of olive oil and a glass of wine. Most of the foods involved include fruits, fish, vegetables, and whole grains.

The Mediterranean Diet features:

- Replacing salt with herbs and spices
- Eating plant-based diets
- Eating fish and skinless chicken twice a week
- Using olive oil and canola to cook
- Drinking wine in moderation
- Exercising

With this diet, you should avoid added sugars, Trans fats, processed meats like sausages, and refined grains.

Benefits of Mediterranean Diet

It is low in sugar and processed foods

Unlike most American diets, the Mediterranean diet consists mainly of natural ingredients, e.g., olive oil, unrefined cereals, fruits, and peas. It is also low in refined sugar and also free from genetically modified foods. The good thing about this diet is you don't need to add any artificial flavors and spices.

Yes, most of the people in the Mediterranean region are not vegetarians. However, the diet still calls for limited consumption of meat and meat products helping to make it a more balanced diet.

The Mediterranean diet also promotes weight loss

Eating the Mediterranean diet will help you to lose weight naturally. The diet promotes intake of nutrient-rich foods while limiting the absorption of fat. Fish and most of the dairy products recommended in the diet contain fatty acids that are essential to your body. These nutrients make you feel fuller longer which in turn helps in regulating your blood sugar and manage your body weight.

It also gives you a healthy heart

Omega-3 foods and the monounsaturated fats have been linked to reduced heart disease. Alpha-linoleic acid from the olive oil helps to decrease blood pressure. Nitric oxide contained in olive oil lowers the risk of hypertension. It also helps to improve the endothelial function and promote oxidation in the body.

It improves your mood

Mediterranean diets can also boost your memory and improve your general mood.

Ketogenic diets

The ketogenic diet focuses on high-fat, low-carbohydrate, and adequate protein. The primary purpose of the diet is to burn the fat in your body to provide energy instead of carbohydrates.

Carbohydrates are usually converted to glucose by the liver for easy absorption. When the glucose level is too high, it increases the level of blood sugar. But, when you are on a low-carbohydrate diet, your body will convert the fats stored in ketone bodies and fatty acids to be used as fuel.

Even though the diet has been used as a medicine especially for epileptic children, people seeking to lose weight can benefit from this diet too.

With the ketogenic diet, you need to plan ahead somewhat for meals so that you can have something ready to eat when you need it. You should aim to attain ketosis (elevated levels of ketone bodies). What you eat will determine how fast you will enter the ketosis stage.

The ketogenic diet focuses on taking in limited amounts of carbohydrates. So, you will need to avoid refined carbs (bread, cereals, and pasta), fruit, and starch (legumes, beans, and potatoes)

You should focus your attention on eating meat (eggs, lean meat, lamb, poultry, and fish), green vegetables, nuts, avocado, berries, macadamia, and olive oil.

How to Attain Ketogenic Diet

Limit your carbohydrate intake

If you want to be successful in this diet, you need to limit your intake to 35g or less of total carbs per day.

Lower your protein intake

To achieve weight loss; you should limit your intake to 0.8 g per pound.

Focus on the fat

Fat is the main energy source in a ketone diet, so you need to eat more of it.

Be sure to drink plenty of water

This is important to keep your body hydrated at all times. Water helps to maintain the normal functioning of your body.

Benefits of Ketogenic Diet

Weight loss

The ketogenic diet will aid in weight loss as it burns the body fat as energy. A ketogenic diet has produced better weight loss results for most people than the low-carb diets.

Helps in controlling blood cholesterol and pressure

Ketogenic diet helps to elevate the triglycerides levels in the body which are linked to the buildup in the arteries.

The ketogenic diet improves insulin sensitivity

Research shows that a ketogenic diet can help in reducing the level of insulin in the blood.

Side effects

Diabetic ketoacidosis

This is a life-threatening diabetic complication. The condition is triggered by elevated levels of the ketone bodies in the blood. High level of the ketone bodies is accompanied by hypoglycemia, insulin deficiency, and dehydration. Symptoms of diabetic ketoacidosis include confusion, vomiting, gasping for breath, increased urination, and abdominal pain. You may also develop bad breath.

DKA is mostly experienced by people with type I diabetes but can occur in other types of diabetes in exceptional circumstances.

If you have diabetes, don't try this diet without your doctor's go ahead.

Cramps

As you start off the diet, you will experience cramps, especially on your legs. The leg cramps will occur due to lack of essential minerals (magnesium). You can experience pain your legs during the morning and also at nights. It is important to include salt in your food to lower the loss of magnesium. You also need to be sure to drink plenty of water.

Constipation

Dehydration causes constipation. You also need to add fiber-rich vegetables in your diet to promote healthy bowel movement.

Reduced levels of energy

You will experience low energy levels when you start using the diet. Your activity level will also reduce.

Atkins Diet

Atkins diet is a fad diet, but it has shown to be an effective tool when it comes to weight loss.

The diet is named after its creator Robert C. Atkins. The Atkins diet focus on restricting carbohydrate intake while increasing the intake of protein and fats. According to cardiologist Robert, obesity results from a low-fat, but high-carbohydrate diet. So, to reduce the weight loss, one must focus on balancing out the protein and fats.

The Atkins diet does not require you to count your calories or even focus on portion control. It advocates people to watch what type of carbohydrates they eat on a daily basis. You need to pay attention to your intake of net carbohydrates (total carbohydrates less fiber content)

While the diet doesn't advocate for weight loss, you should incorporate workout routines in your life for effective results.

Four phases of Atkins Diet

The induction phase

This is phase one, and it requires you to cut down all your carbohydrate intake from your diet. Replace the carbohydrate calories by eating vegetables. You need to increase your consumption of protein (fish, eggs, cheese, meat, and poultry). You should avoid pasta, bread, nuts, grains, baked goods, and most fruits. Drinking at least eight glasses of water per day is essential

Balancing phase

It is phase two which involves slowly adding back the nutrient-rich carbohydrates. In this stage, you will continue to take 12 to 15gm of net carbs. It is recommended you stay in phase two until you attain a weight loss of 10 pounds.

Pre-maintenance (phase three)

You gradually increase the types of food you consume. You will begin to include fruits, and whole grain, and starchy vegetables into your diet. You are allowed to add 10gm of carbohydrates into your diet each week. If the weight loss stops, cut back on the carbs.

Lifetime maintenance (phase four)

You will move to this stage once you attain your ideal weight.

Benefits of Atkins Diet

- ✓ Weight loss
- ✓ Reduces cravings to sweets
- ✓ Increased control of the blood sugar level
- ✓ Low risk of heart disease (not in all cases)
- ✓ Enhanced brain function
- ✓ Reduced risk of some types of cancer
- ✓ Lowers the level of cholesterol in the body
- ✓ Helps in the treatment of PCOS (Polycystic Ovarian Syndrome)

Side effects

Yes, the Atkins diet helps to increase weight loss. However, the diet comes with a set of problems. You may experience fatigue, lethargy, insomnia, constipation, mood swings (caused by low levels of serotonin levels), bad breath, and loss of interest in activities.

Vegetarian diet

Vegetarian diets have become popular over the last couple of decades because of their benefits. Not only do the diets lower the risk of heart disease, but they also aid in weight loss and reduce the risk of diabetes. You can be either a full vegetarian or partial vegetarian.

Different Varieties of Vegetarian Diet

Lacto-vegetarian

This diet excludes the consumption of eggs, poultry, fish, and meat. You can, however, include dairy products like butter, cheese, milk, or yogurt.

Lacto-Ovo vegetarian diet

With this diet, you will eliminate meat, poultry, and fish, but include eggs and dairy products.

Ovo-vegetarian

This diet does not include seafood, poultry, meat, and dairy products. They do, however, include eggs.

Pescatarian diet

With this diet, you can eat fish, but eliminate eggs, dairy, meat, and poultry.

Strict vegetarian (vegan)

You eliminate all the dairy products, eggs, fish, poultry, meat, and all their associated products.

Benefits of Vegetarian Diet

The vegetarian diets are high in antioxidants

Plant-based foods contain a significant amount of antioxidants that help in slowing down the aging process. The vegetarian diet also contains anti-inflammatory properties which help to stop the progression of diseases.

Because they are so rich in nutrients, the vegetarian diets help to boost your immunity and also improve your overall health.

It can help in weight loss

Consuming vegetables and fruits will help you in cutting down on the unwanted pounds. Vegetables are rich in fiber which makes you feel fuller for longer. This will eventually reduce your food intake.

A vegetarian diet improves overall heart health

Taking in vegetables in plenty reduces inflammation (which causes heart diseases). Because of the fiber content in the vegetables and fruits, you will reduce the overall cholesterol levels in your body.

The only real drawback is that a vegetarian diet will put you at an increased risk of micronutrient deficiencies. You may have to take nutrient supplements to meet your daily requirement.

When you are planning your meals, it is essential that you focus on the eating adequate amounts of proteins.

The South Beach Diet

Cardiologist Arthur Agatston created this diet in 2003, is a modified low-carb diet. The primary goal of the South Beach diet is not only to promote weight loss but also improve your overall health.

The diet is low in carbohydrates, but not as low as the low-carb diets. In the South Beach diet, you can get 28% of your total calories from the carbohydrates.

Three phases of the South Beach Diet

Phase one

The purpose of this phase is to eliminate your food cravings. The phase should last for about two weeks. In this phase, you eat lean meat, high-fiber vegetables, skinless chicken, soy products, seafood, avocados, and nuts.

Phase two

You begin to gradually add back into your diet specific foods like whole-grains and pasta, brown rice, more vegetables, and fruits. Phase two is a long-term phase, and you should stay on it until you attain your weight loss goal.

Phase three

It is the maintenance phase where you continue to use the principles provided for a healthy life. You can eat all types of food but in moderation.

Benefits of South Beach Diet

- ✓ South beach diet aids in weight loss
- ✓ Help to reduce hunger and provide satiety
- ✓ It helps to fight inflammation

Even though the diet is beneficial to most people, it promotes the intake of vegetable oils which contain Trans fats.

Every diet is unique and will have a different effect on your body. It is, therefore, very important for you to consult your doctor before choosing a diet.

Chapter 7:
Exercises to Help You Lose Weight

Attaining your ideal body weight is not a walk in the park. You need a proper diet and more so exercises that are tailored towards helping you achieve your weight loss goal. Understanding the impact each set of workout routines has on your body is essential for you.

Before you can design a workout routine, you need first to know your end goals. Do you want to lose weight or simply build muscle and strength? Secondly, you need to understand your body type. We all have different body types with distinct features. Not every exercise is going to be suitable for you.

Three Body Types

Ectomorph

People with this body type tend to be thin and lean and often struggle to gain either muscle or body weight.

Though they may appear thin and weak, they have body strength. As an ectomorph, you need to be careful what you eat. Most people think that even with this body type you can just eat what you want. However, it is not only weight that can put your health at risk. Keep in mind that not all people who have diabetes are overweight.

Mesomorph

As a mesomorph, you will have a narrow waist, broad shoulder, and thin joints. People with this body type tend to lose weight relatively quickly.

Endomorph

If you have this body type, you will gain weight and keep it. Your body will appear wider than the mesomorph as you have wider hips and shorter limbs. With this body type, you have more muscles, but you will struggle to build them up as you also have body fat.

Once you understand which category you belong to, it will be easy to design a workout plan that will help you burn the body fat and also build your muscles.

General weight loss exercises

Cardio exercises

Regardless of your body type, a good regime of cardio exercises are essential. They play a significant role in the health of your heart. Remember, your heart is also a muscle, and just like your body muscles, it needs exercise. Cardio exercises are designed to increase your general heart rate. Aerobics use your leg muscles.

As you are working out, your heart rate should be increased, but you should be able to breathe normally. If you can't talk to other people while you are working out, it is an indication you are working too hard.

Significant Benefits of Cardio Exercises

- ✓ They promote burning of calories
- ✓ The practices increase your heart rate and function
- ✓ You will enjoy an improved lung function
- ✓ The exercises help to improve the cholesterol and the triglyceride levels in the body
- ✓ They help to reduce osteoporosis

- ✓ You will enjoy better sleep and mental capacity
- ✓ Cardio workouts trigger the production of the endorphins

The duration of the cardio exercises will differ based on your goals. If you want to burn fat, you should perform one exercise routine for more than 30 minutes. Your body will begin to burn the body fat after 30 minutes of exercise. You should, however, ensure you don't go past 60 minutes as it will increase your risk of injury.

The frequency of the exercises should be limited to at least four times a week for best results.

Walking

Walking is perfect for people who are starting out. Walking is a simple exercise that can be done anywhere. You need the right walking shoes. You should also avoid wearing tight workout clothes as they may interfere with blood flow.

It is vital for you to avoid walking in direct sun exposure as you will end up feeling tired. The best time to hike is in the morning. You may also need a work out partner to keep you motivated. Be sure that you always drink plenty of water while hiking.

Cycling

Cycling is one of the few exercises that help you burn fat and also builds your muscle. For the advanced cyclists, using a mountain bike is perfectly fine. However, if you are just getting started, you can opt for stationary bikes as they will give the same effect.

Elliptical exercises

To perform these exercises, you will need the elliptical trainer. It is a stationary machine that mimics stair climbing. You can walk and run at the same time on an elliptical machine. The equipment helps you to exercise without the risk of injuries or damaging your joints. Another advantage is that you work your upper body as well as you're lower.

Swimming

Swimming is perfect for you if you don't like working out in the gym. With this exercise, you will use both your upper and lower body muscles. Swimming targets your core, arms, glutes, back, and legs. You can use different swimming techniques to achieve better results.

Jumping rope exercises

If you are looking for an efficient yet affordable exercise routine, jump rope exercises are perfect. These activities are simple and can be done in the comfort of your own home. Even though using a jumping rope is simple, you need to wear protective workout clothes especially the shoes to ease impact your joints.

Stair climber exercises

Several stair climber types are available in two options, a stepper (they come with a pedal) or a rolling stair (they are designed with rolling stairs). Stair climbing exercises will help you to tone your muscles as well as burn fat. The best thing about these exercises is that they will work all your leg muscles.

Rowing exercises

Rowing exercises are done with the help of a rowing machine. The exercises benefit both your lower and upper body. Adding rowing exercises to your workout routine will help you burn fat as well as tone your body.

HIIT

The High-Intensity Interval Training exercise is a whole-body workout. The exercises will promote weight loss as well as tone your muscles. The HIIT exercises differ greatly depending on the number of calories that you seek to burn. You can burn 500 calories to about 1500 calories per hour depending on the exercise that you choose.

The HIIT is great because they combine bodyweight movement with muscle building exercises.

Kettlebells

The kettlebells exercises may not necessarily be a cardio exercise, but they help in burning calories. These exercises combine cardio as well as strength training.

Sprinting

Regardless of where you choose to sprint whether, on a treadmill, outside, or on bleachers, you can be guaranteed that you will lose weight. One advantage of these exercises is that they do not require any equipment.

Sprinting involves simple moves, but they help burn a large number of calories. Because of its simple techniques, the sprint exercise should not cause any injury to your muscles.

Jogging

Jogging at a moderate pace can help burn fat. Jogging is a great cardio workout however it may not help you to build your muscles.

Stretching and balance exercises

Stretching helps to improve your flexibility and also strengthen your muscles. These exercises if done correctly will help to prevent injuries while working out. Stretching will also help to reduce back pain. Stretched muscles improve your body movement and performance.

There are different stretching and balancing exercises that you can choose to engage in.

Yoga

Yoga has been used for many decades now to promote flexibility. The different poses have improved the general mood and promote mental clarity. One of the biggest benefits of yoga that people often do not realize is that it helps you lose weight. Performing the different poses will help you to burn your body fat. Before you can begin yoga, you need to consult a yoga master or practitioner. They will provide you with guidance about which of the different yoga poses that you can engage in safely.

Pilates

Pilates, just like yoga focuses on improving the body strength by emphasizing on core strength and flexibility. Pilate exercises benefit the whole body. These exercises are also adaptable and can be used by just about anybody.

Pilates doesn't focus on flexibility alone, it also aids in weight loss, and will help you to improve your muscle tone. The different poses which make up the Pilates exercise will help to improve your posture.

Pilate exercises come in various moves that you can try.

Swimming

With this move, you lie on your stomach. You lift your forehead and pubis. Make sure that there is a fist-length between your neck and chin. Your arms should be stretched, and your inner thighs pressed together. Alternate the movement of your feet and arms. It is essential for you to inhale and exhale while you exercise (your muscles need the oxygen)

Crisscross

The move requires you to lie on your back. Your head should be lifted and your arms layered on the back of the head. You will lift your left knee to connect with your right elbow and vice versa. Continue with the technique until you attain the required number of sets.

Leg Pull

Extend your legs as you are seated. Place your palms down and elevate your hips until you attain a diagonal line. Lift your leg as high as it can go without you shifting your body.

Corkscrew

You will have to lie down on your mat with your arms extended on the side. Lift your legs slowly overhead until you balance the middle part of your shoulder with the back of your arms. Make sure you inhale slowly.

Tai Chi

Tai Chi promotes flexibility, reduces levels of stress, lowers blood pressure, promotes better sleep, and aids in weight loss among other benefits. The exercises involve simple movements and thus make it suitable for most people. Before you can begin the exercises, you need to warm up. The different Tai Chi movements include;

Windmill exercises

These moves help to protect your spine as well as promote flexibility.

Hand exercises

These help to improve the movement and flexibility of your arms, fingers, and shoulders.

Knee rolls

These exercises will help to improve flexibility in your knees and spine.

Closing posture

These moves are done at the end of the Tai chi exercises.

Strength training

It is not only about weight loss, but you also need to build your overall body strength to enable you to perform your daily activities.

Benefits of Strength Training

- ✓ The exercises will help you to maintain your weight loss
- ✓ The exercises help you to protect both your muscle mass and bone health
- ✓ You will feel stronger and also helps improves your mood
- ✓ The exercises promote better body coordination, posture, and flexibility

- ✓ These exercises help in the management of arthritis and also prevent the occurrence of disease
- ✓ Strength training exercises help to improve your general health. It reduces the risk of diabetes and cardiovascular diseases.

Simple Principles Adhered on Strength Exercises

Type of strength training

You should choose an exercise based on your specific body needs. Use the specific exercises and equipment to target your work out area of interest.

Intensity

It refers to the amount of effort that you put in every exercise.

Variety

To achieve better results, use a variety of exercise in each set. Different exercises will affect your muscles differently forcing them to adapt.

Volume

What is the duration of your workouts? You can increase or decrease the length based on your goals.

Rest

It is crucial for you to rest in between sets.

Increase your work out weights

Gradually increasing your workout weights will make your muscles to build up and grow stronger

Recover

You will need to set time off to recover. Your muscles need to repair themselves after every workout. You should rest for at least 48 hours.

Barbell exercises

Barbell exercises require barbells and their associated weight plates. To perform these exercises, you will need a good quality bench press. It is crucial for you to be cautious when you are working out with the barbells. Your body has not yet adjusted or stabilized. Maintaining good posture while working out is essential to avoid any injuries.

Dumbbell exercises

Unlike other exercises, dumbbell exercises do not isolate specific muscles. To efficiently workout, you will need to use almost all of your muscles. You will require a set of dumbbells to workout. The dumbbells are available in different sizes. You can either get the fixed weight or adjustable dumbbells (allow you to adjust the weight every time you work out).

The risk of bodily injury is high with these dumbbell exercises, so be careful. You need to exercise caution and also maintain the right posture, and it might be a good idea to have a friend spot you why you exercise.

Chapter 8:

Getting in the Right Mindset to Maintain Healthy Diabetes Levels

Maintaining your diabetes is not only about following the doctor's direction, you need to have the right mindset to follow through with the program that you choose to try to control your diabetes. It takes a lot of mental preparation and motivation for you to succeed in any weight loss and exercise program that you choose.

Most people start off their program with a lot of enthusiasm, but as days go by, their motivation starts to diminish. Lack of Willpower will force them to go back to your old eating habits and if you are diabetic, you can't afford to mess with your diet.

How to prepare mentally

So, how can you ensure you prepare yourself mentally for the journey ahead?

Get a dietician

Before you can begin your weight loss journey, you should consult a registered dietician. They will help you to choose a diet suitable for your health needs. The dietician should also follow up with you after your sessions to monitor your progress.

You might also consider enrolling in a gym that caters to people with diabetes.

Set your goals

Taking the time to write down your weight loss goals will help you to develop an action plan. Not setting clear goals will be a roadblock in your progress.

- ✓ Setting goals will give you focus
- ✓ Specific goals will help you to measure your progress, however small it may be
- ✓ Goals will help you to overcome procrastination
- ✓ Smart goals will give you motivation

You can follow the S.M.A.R.T method while setting your goals;

Specific

The goals you set should be specific to your situation. Writing down your goal as weight loss is vague and not as motivating. You should include the number of pounds that you want to lose in a specified period.

Measurable

You should be able to track the number of calories or pounds that you have lost.

Achievable

Setting unrealistic goals will lead to failure. It is understandable for you to be enthusiastic about losing weight, but wanting to lose 25 pounds in two weeks is unrealistic. Keep in mind that a 'journey of a thousand miles begins with one step.' Setting small goals that are achievable will keep you motivated to continue.

Realistic

Do not set vague over the top goals

Time-bound

Every goal that you set should have a period for when you will achieve it. Having a time frame will help you to eliminate all the distractions that might be present. Avoid giving yourself an unrealistic time frame.

Dieticians recommend a weight loss of 2 to 4 pounds per week. So, your goals should be per the recommendations. Keep in mind that losing your weight too fast can be harmful to your health.

Mental visualization

Mental visualization is the best way to reprogram your subconscious mind. Have a picture of how you will look at the end. When you view it in your mind, it will be only a matter of time before you see it manifest in your body.

Creating a vision board is a great way to visualize your goals. If you had photos of yourself when you were on your ideal weight, stick them on the vision board. You can also take a picture or buy a dress that is one size smaller and hang it on your vision board. This way you will have a view before you of what goal you want to achieve.

It is recommended that you hang your vision board somewhere visible so it can be easy for you to remember your goals.

Have a detailed plan

Create an action plan of how you will get from where you are, to where you want to be. The action plan should include the type of exercises that you want to engage in. You also need to include what kind of diet that you want to try. If you have a meal plan, include it in your action plan.

Write down all the steps you will take to ensure that you are following the right track.

Get support

Having someone hold you accountable is essential. Talk to your family members about your plan and ask them for their support. They will help you to stay on the right course for your weight loss program.

Positive affirmations

Your body will maintain your new lifestyle if your mind is comfortable with it. Being positive about your process will help your mind to stay motivated. You keep your mind positive with positive affirmations.

Affirmations are how you talk yourself (self-talk). They are statements about yourself and how you view your situation. Do you know you talk to yourself more than you do other people? The problem is some people have a negative self-talk which affects their motivation and their output in life. You can't hope to lose weight and maintain a healthy lifestyle if you always have a negative attitude.

Positive affirmations will help you to stay motivated and focused on your goals. Take time to write down statements that are related to your situation. You can get a few affirmations for weight loss on the internet. Every morning, take a few minutes to speak them out loud. You will be surprised what your mind will do if you have a positive attitude towards your weight loss process.

Replace your bad habits

We are creatures of habits. 90 % of our daily life is carried out because of our practices. Did you know it is easier to form a good habit than it is for you to break a bad one? Psychologists say it takes about 21 days for a person to master a new practice. So, find ways that you can replace your bad habits. For example; if you have a problem with eating candy and drinking sugary items, you can replace them with healthier options like fruits.

Do not focus on forming several new habits at once. Choose one practice and stick with it until you master it and can subconsciously perform it.

Be patient

Weight loss is a long-term process. You need to have patience not only in yourself but also in the diet that you choose. It may be frustrating for you if you don't lose weight as fast as you expected, but don't get disappointed with yourself. It will take time for you to see progress in your body. So, just focus on the fact that you are healthy.

Reward yourself

When you achieve even a small goal with your weight loss plan, you should reward yourself. This will keep you motivated and focused on your other goals.

Developing Self-discipline

Motivation and willpower will help you to get started with your weight loss program. However, to continue working out and eating healthy as you should, you need self-discipline.

There will come a time when you lack the motivation to go on with the process, and at that moment, you need something more to keep on going. Self-discipline is the ability to do what needs to be done even when you don't feel like it. It is about motivating yourself to wake up in the morning to go to the gym when you are too sleepy too.

Self-discipline is the muscle that holds your weight loss program together. It is essential for you to understand the importance self-discipline has on your life. If you have an awareness of the consequences of indiscipline, you will be committed to the process.

Time management

Time management plays an important role in creating a balance for your life. Lack of proper time management will not only affect your output at work and home but also how you work out. If you don't plan your activities properly in the allocated time, you will end up worn out before the day ends. Do you know that being overwhelmed can affect your blood sugar levels? Self-discipline will help you to plan your activities in order of importance. If you want to get more from your day, it is better, to begin with, the most challenging task first.

When it comes to scheduling time for your workout, make time in the morning before you begin your day. You will have control of whatever happens in the morning as opposed to later in the day when you are already tired.

Creates stability

Self-discipline will teach you about responsibility. It will also help you to develop patience and obedience. Because you are disciplined, you will have mental clarity that helps you to have a better perspective of every situation. You will not overreact about a situation you can't do anything about.

Builds inner strength

Doing what you are supposed to do even when you don't feel like it, will help you to build your character. With self-discipline, you will be able to handle any situation or challenge that comes your way. Inner strength and self-discipline are going to be key for you to manage your diabetes diet and exercise plan.

Helps you to control your appetite and cravings

Self-discipline is about knowing the consequences of any action before you engage in it. You will be in a better position of managing your desires because you understand the consequences of your action.

Self-discipline helps to create balance in your life. It is, therefore, essential for you to develop or strengthen your inner character.

How to develop self-discipline

You can never succeed in anything without having self-discipline. There are a few steps that can help you in developing discipline in every area of your life.

Define what you want

What do you want to achieve? What habits do you want to develop? Knowing that will help you to focus your attention on it.

Self-discipline only works if it is directed to something. A diet or an exercise are the perfect things for you to focus on with self-discipline. Once you plan out a routine to help you control your diabetes and lose weight, stick to it no matter what.

What are the changes that you need to make?

Once you have a mental picture of what you want to achieve, you need to write down the changes that you need to adapt or achieve the outcome.

Each goal that you have written down requires a set of behaviors and habits that you must form if you want to be successful. You also need to have clarity on what you need to eliminate in your life.

Find a role model

If you want to lose weight and build your muscles, then maybe you need to find other people with diabetes that have achieved the lifestyle that you want. Learning from them and their experiences will give you the motivation to be able to stay focused on your own program. Your role model can be a person you know or someone you researched on the internet. Take time to learn about what they did and the obstacles they had to overcome to get to where they are.

Identify your habits

If you are obese or overweight, you need to know the habits that got you in that situation in the first place. Write down all the things you did concerning exercise and the foods that you ate. You will have clarity on what you need to change to lose weight.

Identify your triggers

Once you make a list of the foods that you ate, write down your triggers. Are you an emotional eater? Do you like to eat while watching television? Do you sleep eat? Knowing what makes you binge eat is the first step to overcoming the problem. If it is a psychological process, you need to see a doctor or a counselor.

Develop a plan

Have a plan on what you need to do to live a healthy life. Create mini-milestones for every goal that you have written down. Micro goals will give the motivation to work towards your macro-goals.

Accountability

It is important for you to have an accountability partner. But, you also need to raise your standards. Hold yourself accountable for the goals you want to achieve.

Sources of support

Self-discipline, motivation, and self-will are all essential to successfully managing diabetes. But, you will agree that the journey is not easy. That is why seeking help from support groups will help you manage your condition.

Family and friends

People who are surrounded by their family and loved ones are more likely to manage their condition well. So, reaching out to your family will help you live a stress-free life. They, however, need to have the necessary information to assist you in managing diabetes. They will also hold you accountable to what you eat and your general lifestyle.

Support groups

Join a support group. This will give you an opportunity to connect with people who are going through the same situation as you. Members of a support group share with others on the challenges they have encountered and how they solved them.

If you don't know any support groups, you can ask your doctor or dietician about the local diabetic support groups near you.

Your healthcare team

Your doctor, dietician, and other staff members have years of experience, and they know how to manage diabetes.

Take advantage of every opportunity to ask questions about diabetes.

Online communities

The internet has given you access to different forums that you can join. You will get access to various websites that will provide you with information on how well to manage diabetes. You can search for the 'Diabetic Hands Foundation' and connect with like-minded individuals.

Conclusion

Diabetes is a progressive disease, and it has no cure. When it comes, it stays with you. But, there is good news; you can live a successful and fulfilling life with proper management. Yes, diabetes comes with other complications too that can be detrimental to your health and general lifestyle. You can prevent the diabetic complications or delay their progression by regularly testing and managing your blood sugar.

Regardless of the type of diabetes, there are various ways you can manage your blood sugar.

Choose the right diet

Dieticians and doctors have designed a variety of foods that can help you lose weight and maintain a healthy lifestyle. No two diets are alike, and each will have a different outcome. So, take time to do your research on the diets and their effectiveness. You can talk to your dietician on how to choose a suitable diet.

Planning your meals is also an essential part of managing your diabetes. As you know, there are different meal planning systems that you can choose. The plate method is one of the most straightforward techniques that you can use.

Choose the right exercise routine

Diet alone can't do the trick. You need to combine the right form of exercise to help in your weight loss. Cardio exercises are perfect if weight loss is your ultimate goal. Make a point of alternating the cardio workouts to manage your weight and also blood sugar efficiently. If you want to maintain the weight loss, then weight training exercises are essential.

Consider the alternatives

Diabetes can be managed through several available natural therapies. The beauty of taking the natural herbal supplements is they present little or no side effects. Herbal supplements contain natural ingredients that not only help you to lose weight but also to keep most diabetes complications at bay.

Before you take any herbal supplements, you should talk to your doctor especially if you are on insulin.

Physical exercises are other options that you can opt for aside from natural herbs.

Develop self-discipline and the right mindset

Self- discipline is the backbone of your success. Willpower can take you so far, but when you don't feel like doing what is required of you, you need the self-discipline to pull you up.

Developing self-discipline is not as hard as it may sound. It is all about having small achievable goals. Plan your workout routines per your available time.

Having the right mindset will motivate you to achieve your weight goals and also stay on your diet for the long haul.

Don't do it alone

Have a strong support system that will keep you motivated will help you manage your diabetes successfully. Your family is a perfect place to start. However, having a support group will be beneficial to you. Ask your doctor or healthcare team about any local diabetic support groups. Joining other people who have diabetes will help you to realize you are not alone.

The online community can also be a great forum for you to find support.

Printed in Great Britain
by Amazon